May this book
bring you joy
and sweet memories!
Jen Michelle Lin

M000290750

Dear Vada,

A lifetime will never be enough
to express the joy, love, and
wonder of you.

When you were in my belly,
we counted down the days
until we could meet you.

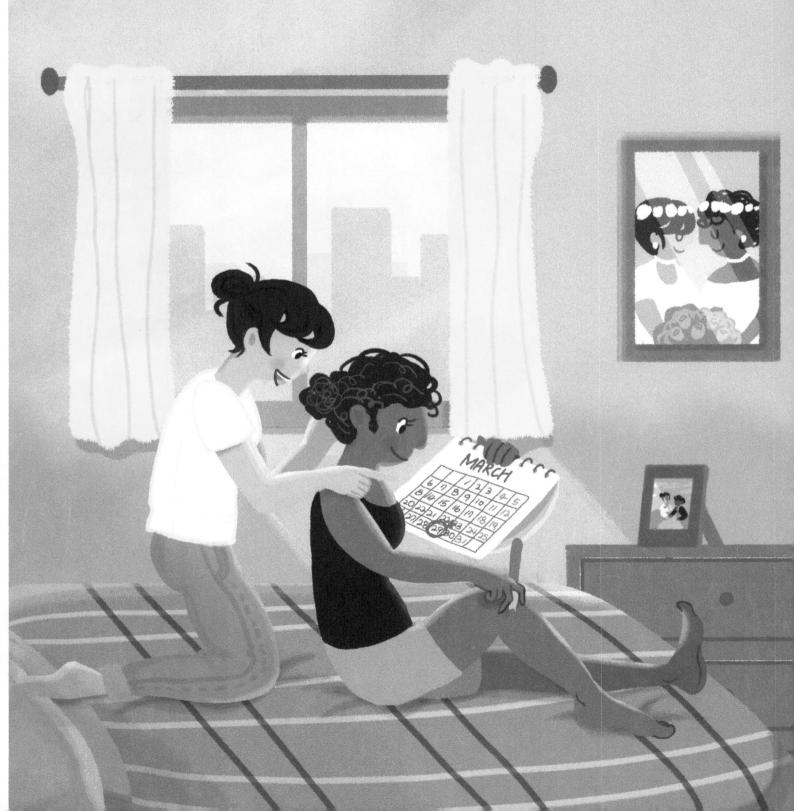

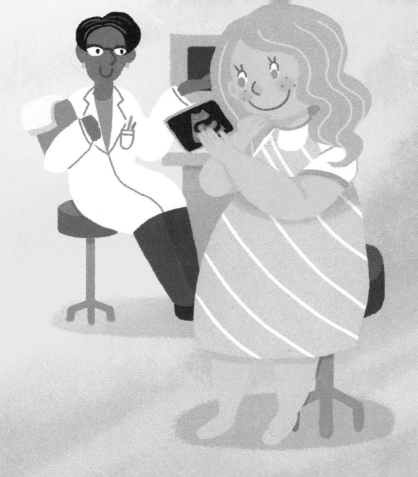

We used each day to plan and prepare for life with you.

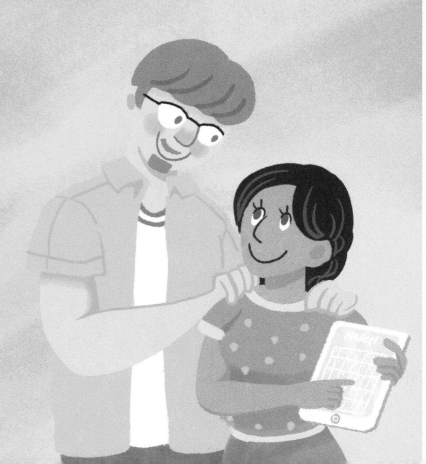

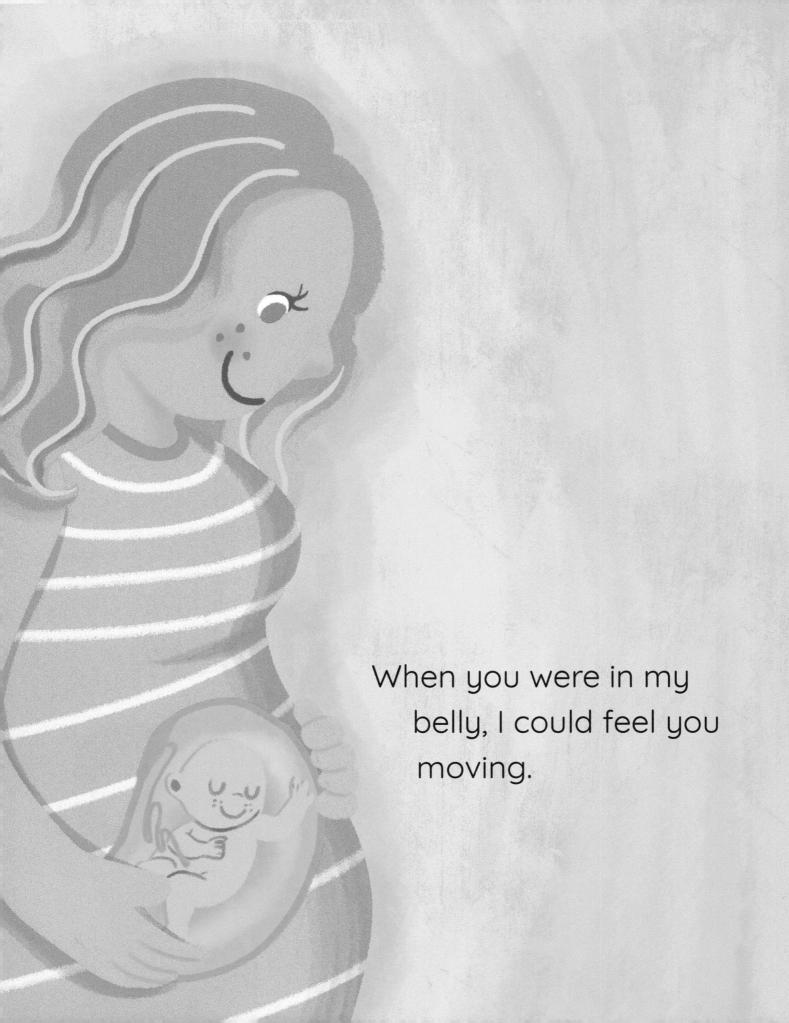

When you were in my belly, I could feel you moving.

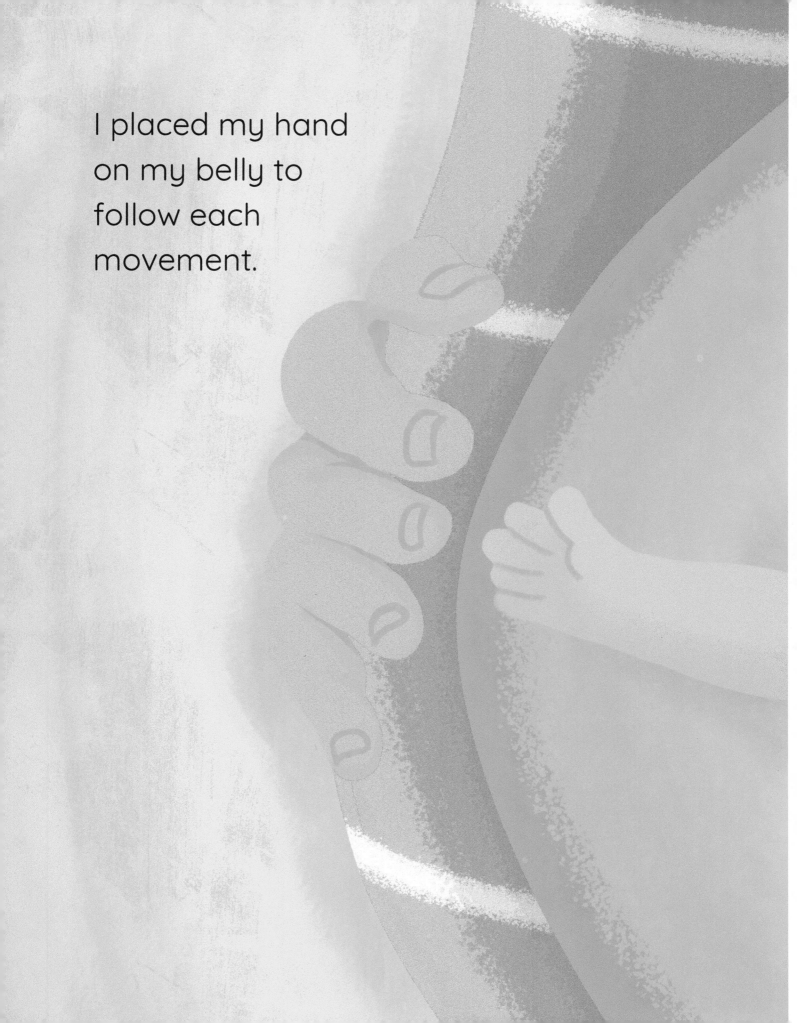

I placed my hand
on my belly to
follow each
movement.

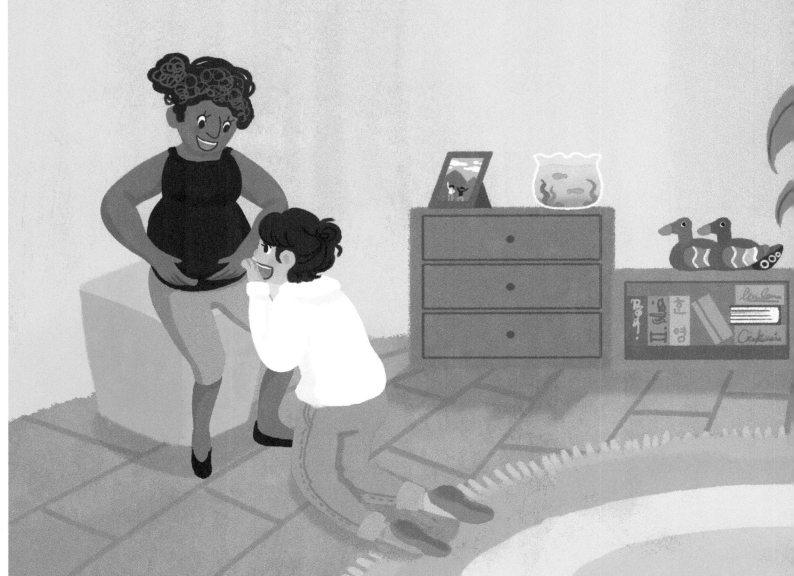

When you
were in my
belly, we spoke
to you so that you
would learn the sounds of our voices.

We played different types of
music to entertain you.

When you were in my belly,
we visited the doctor to listen
to your heartbeat.

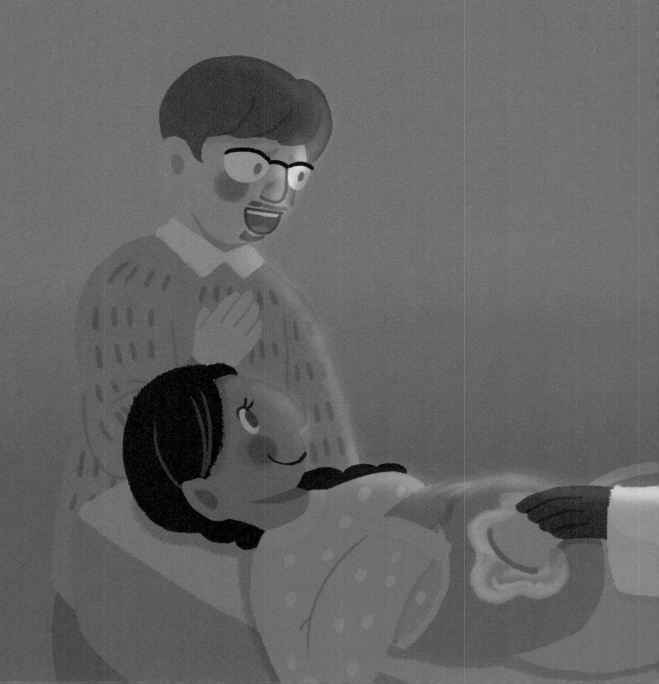

The doctor took pictures of you so we could see your smile and what you were doing.

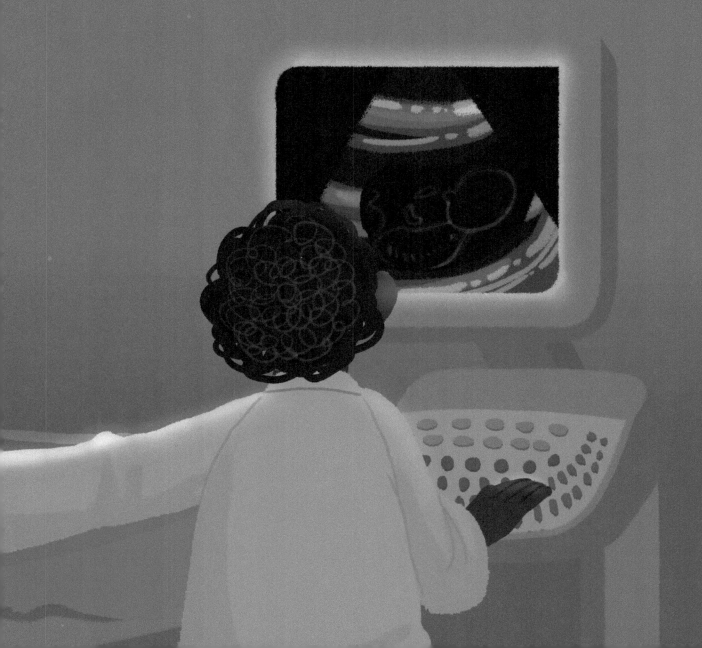

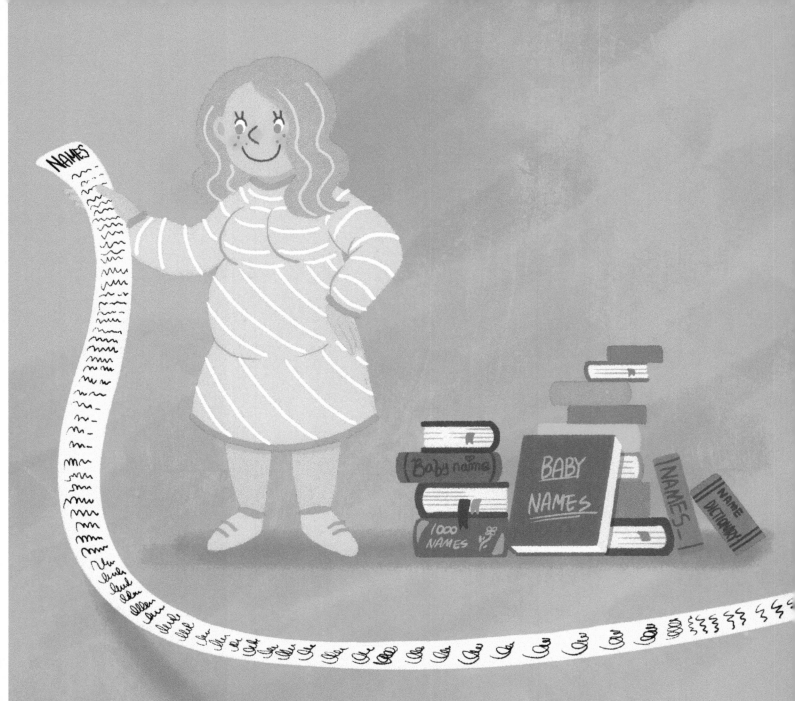

When you were in my belly, we looked through stacks of baby books to search for your name.

We read the meaning of each name, looking for one that meant something special.

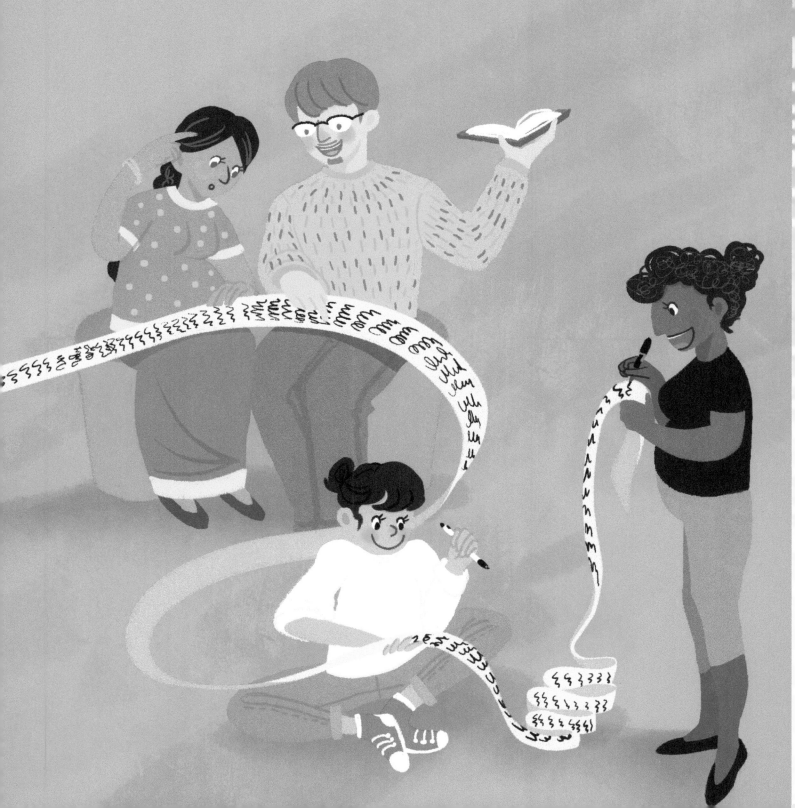

When you were in my belly, we tracked your growth each day.

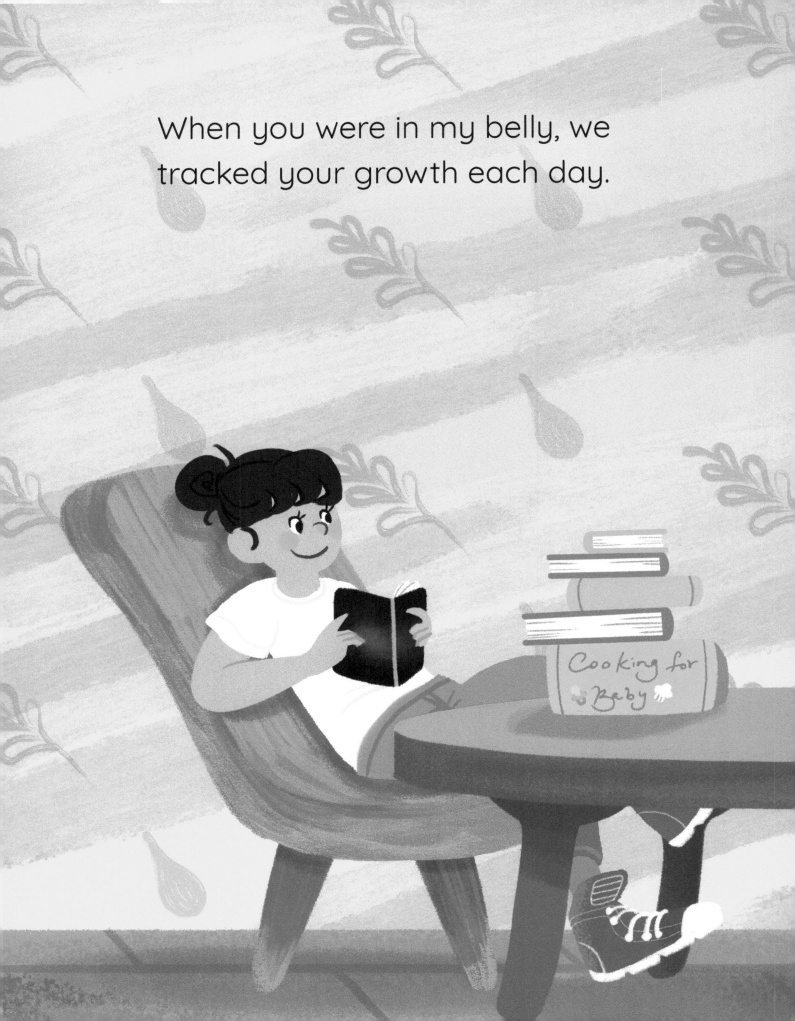

We read books to learn more about how you were growing and what you needed.

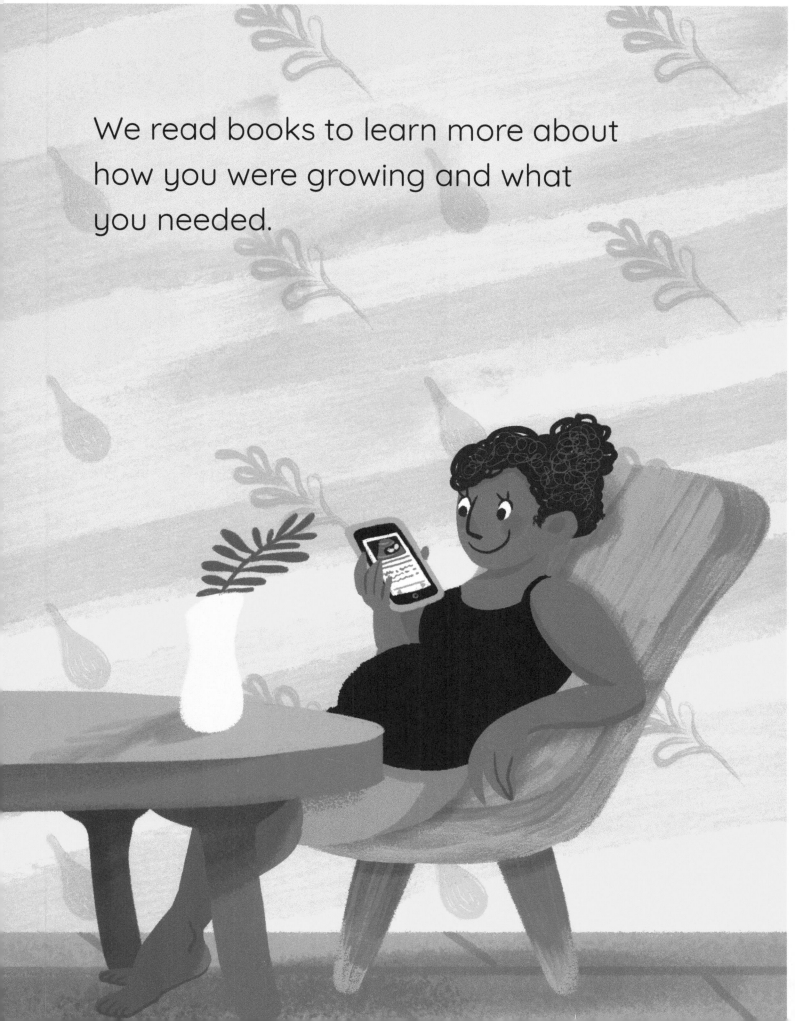

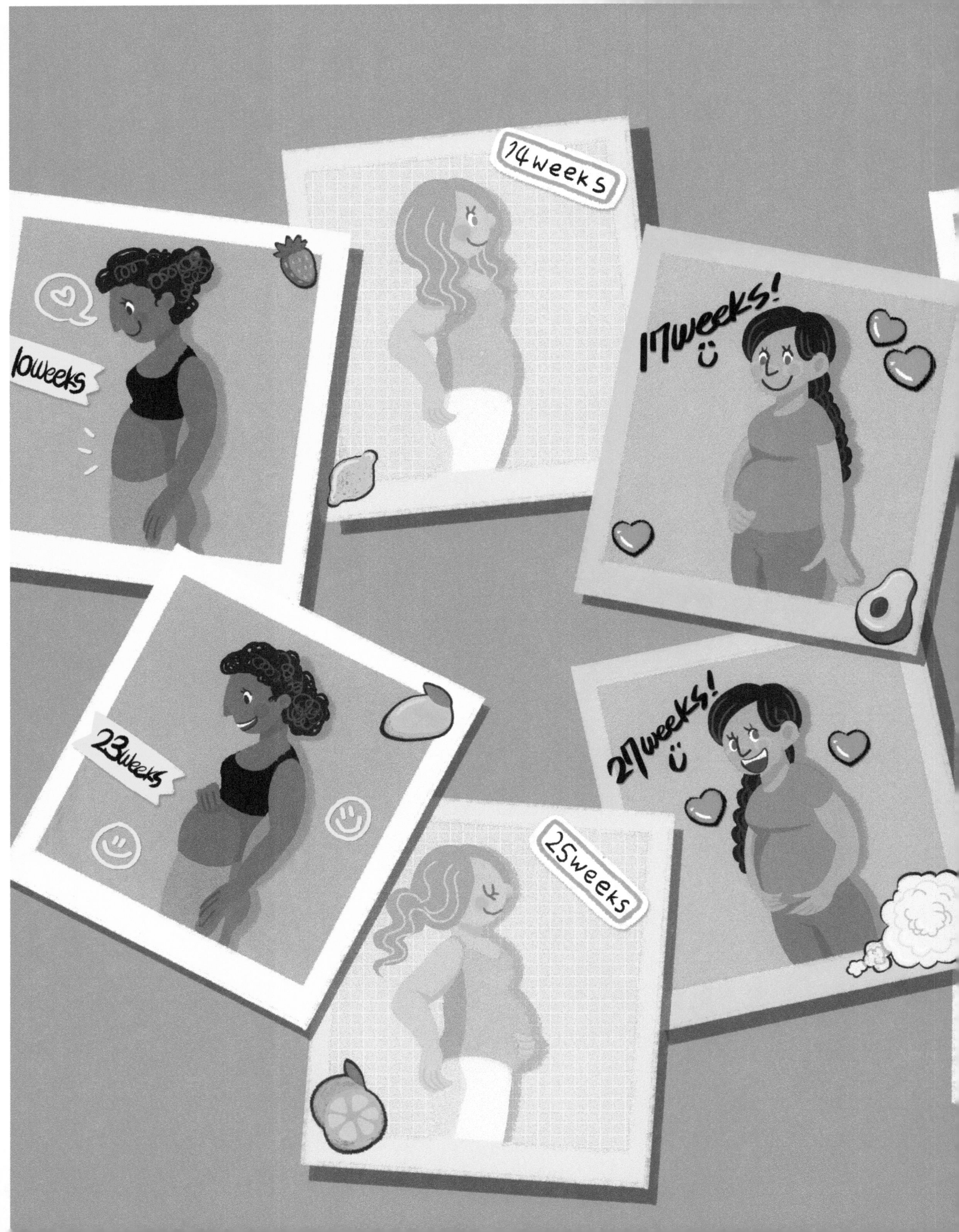
10weeks
14weeks
17weeks!
23weeks
25weeks
27weeks!

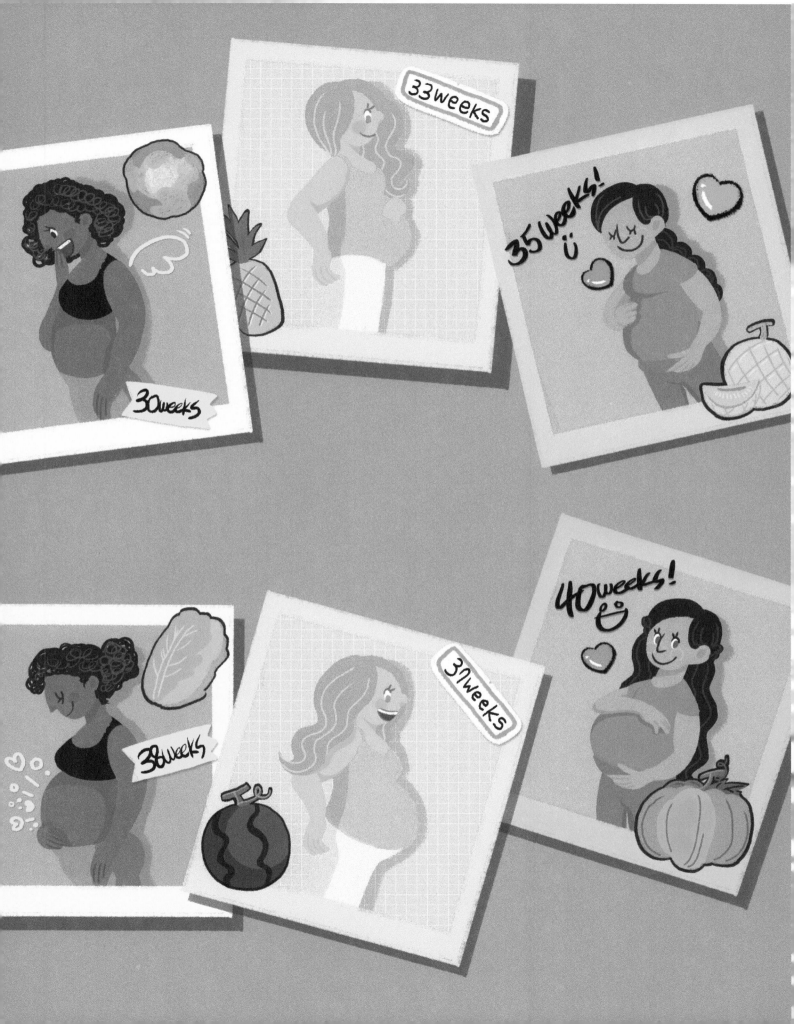

When you were in my belly, I ate plenty of fruits and vegetables to help you grow.

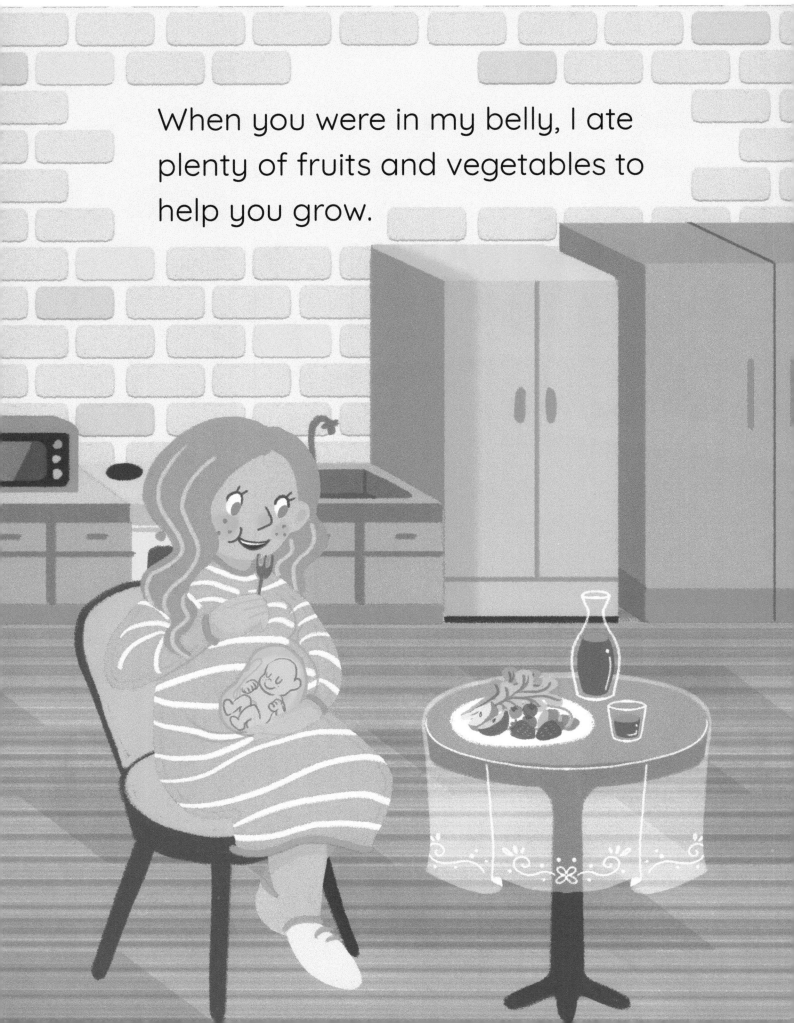

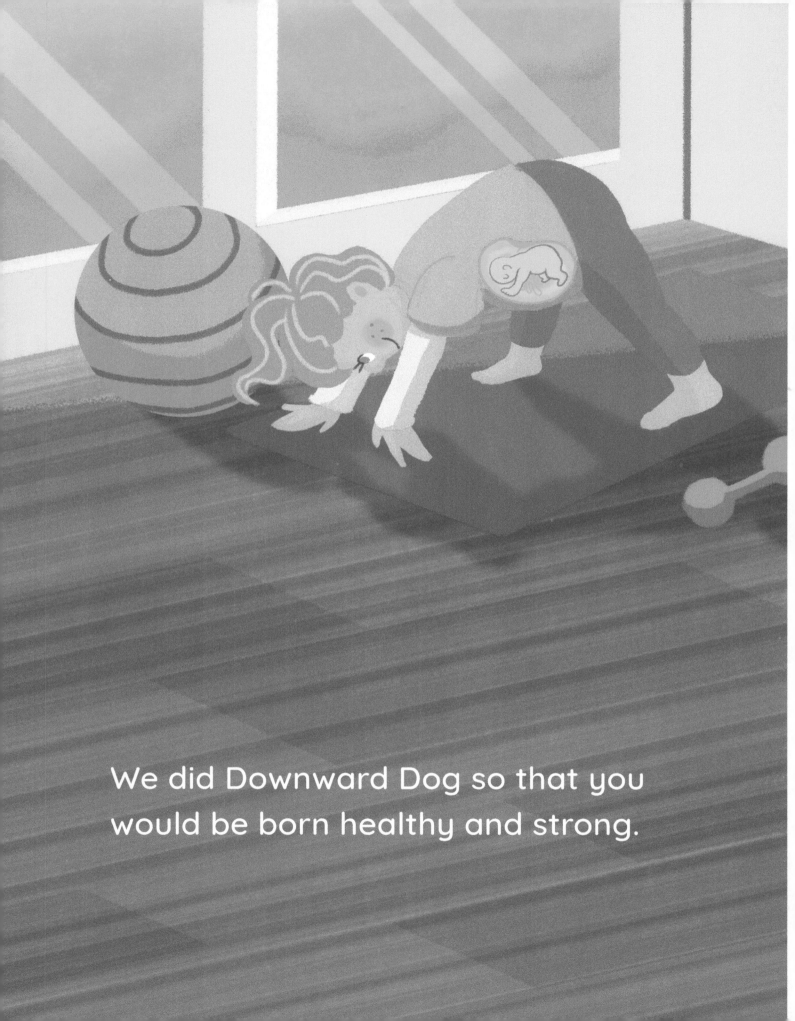

We did Downward Dog so that you would be born healthy and strong.

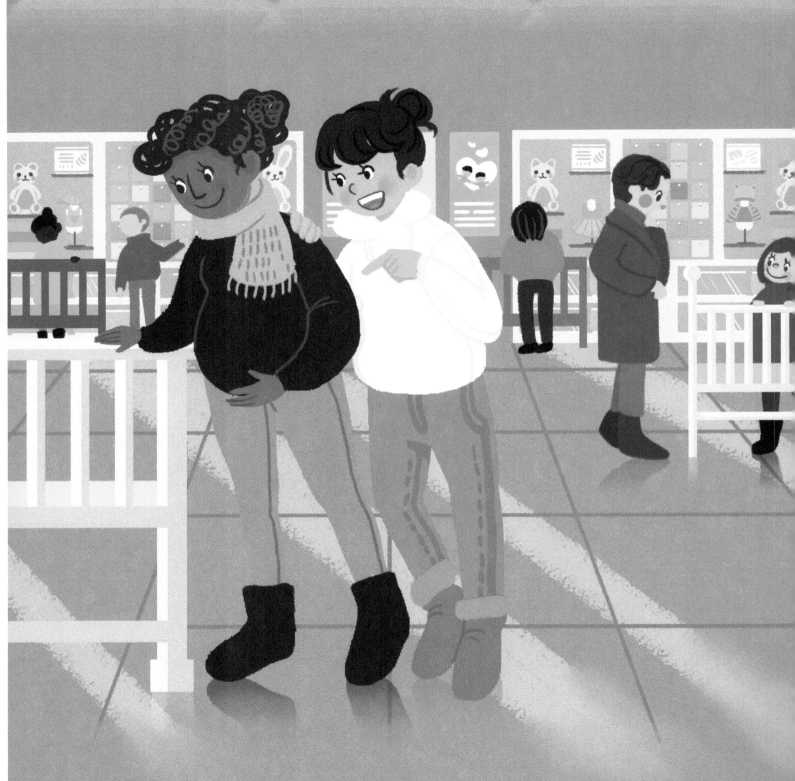

When you were in my belly,
we shopped until we found the
perfect crib for you to sleep in.

We spent hours pushing strollers back and forth to find the best ride.

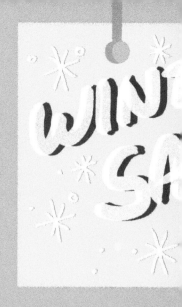

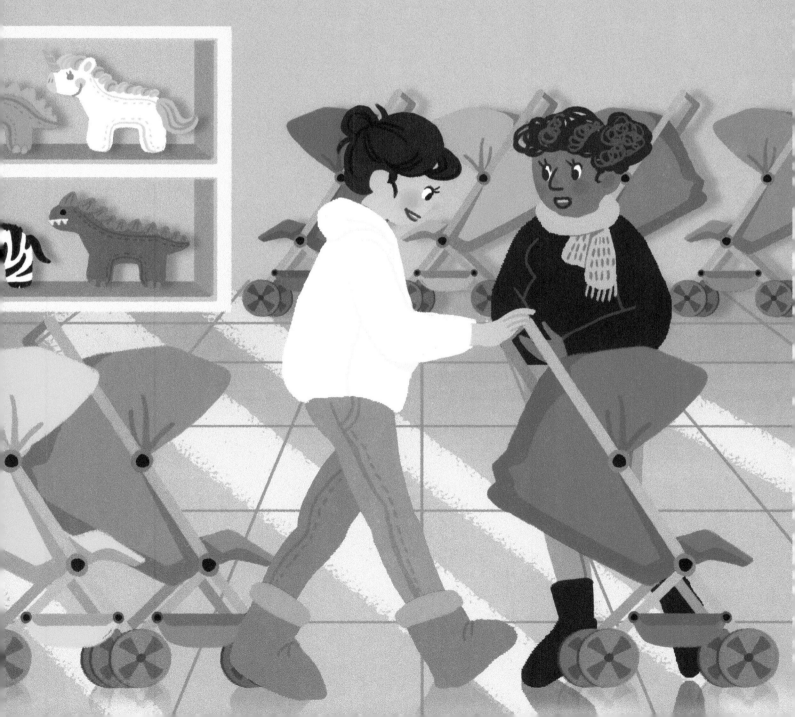

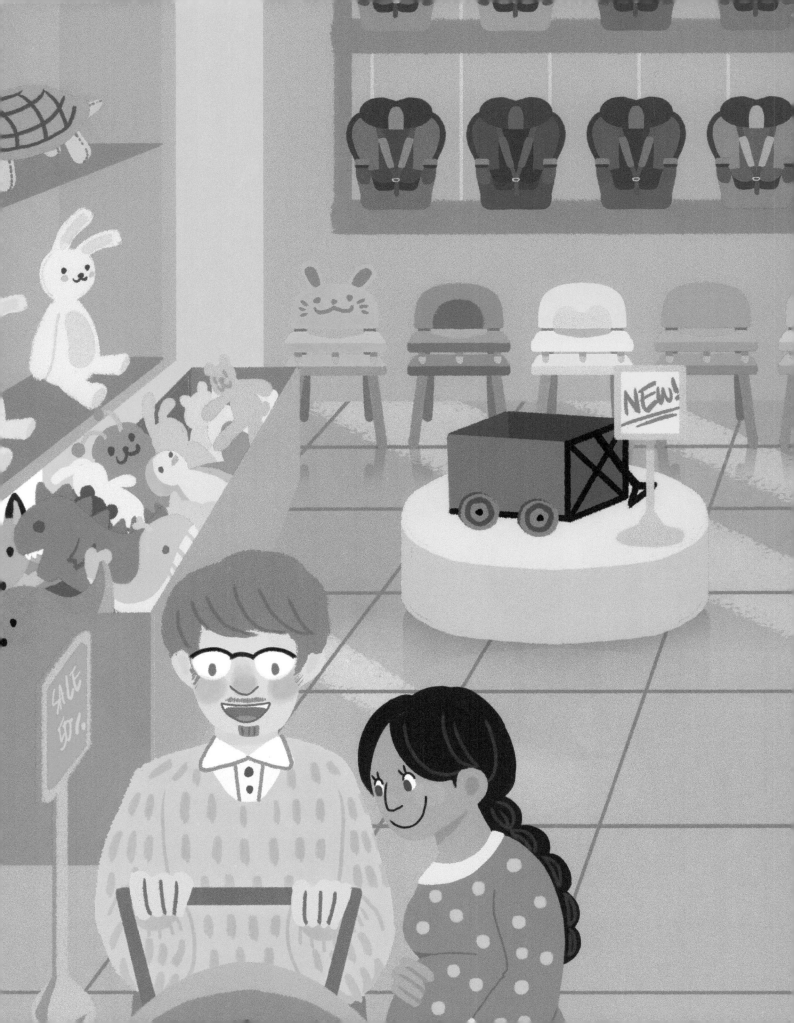

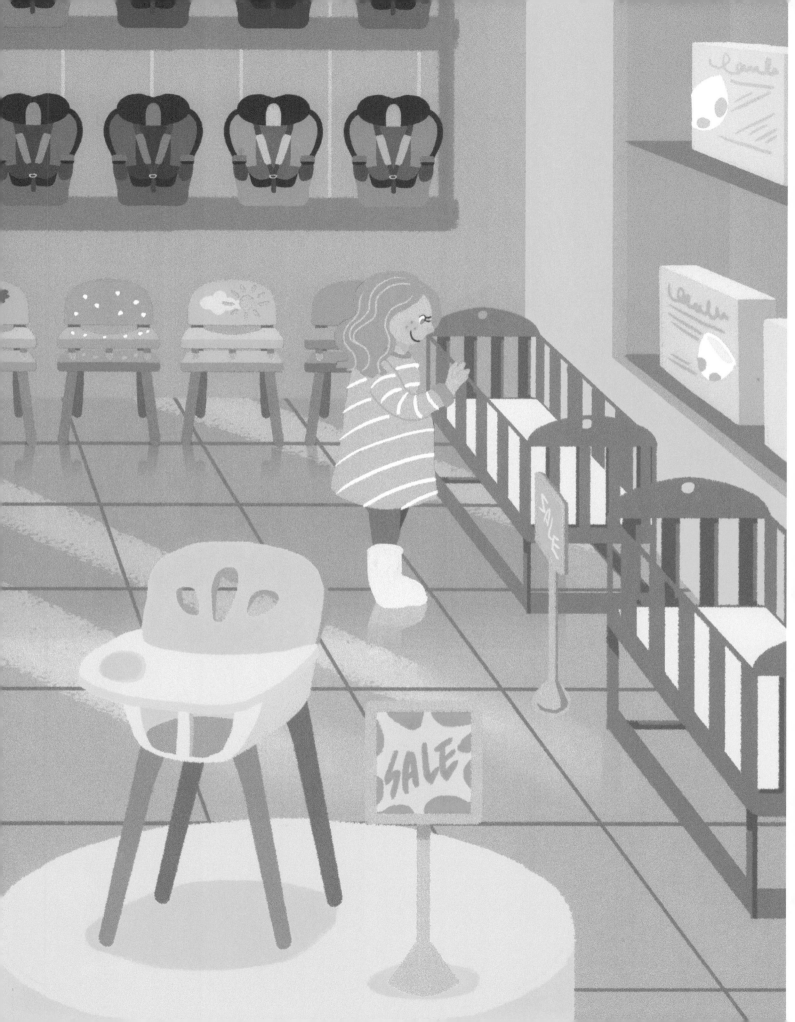

When you were in my belly, we opened gifts from family and friends.

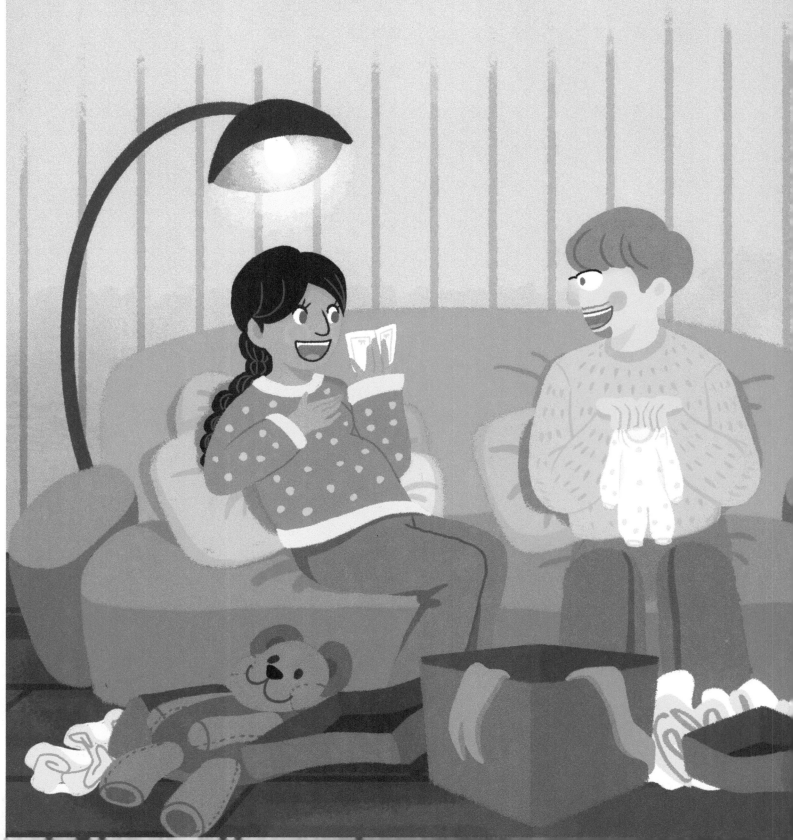

We found places to store all of your clothes and toys.

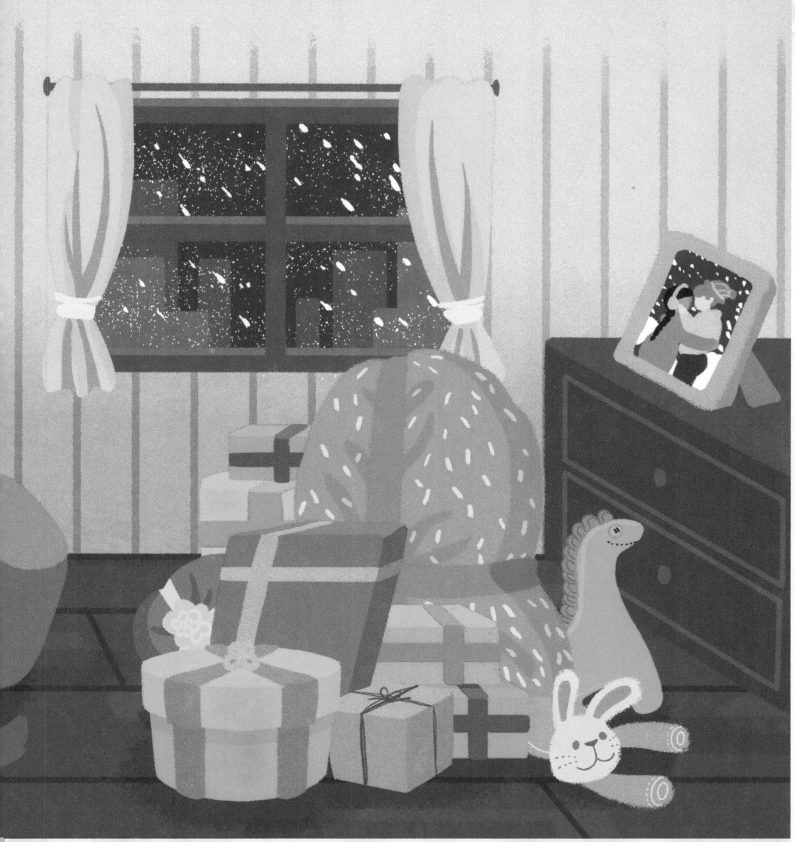

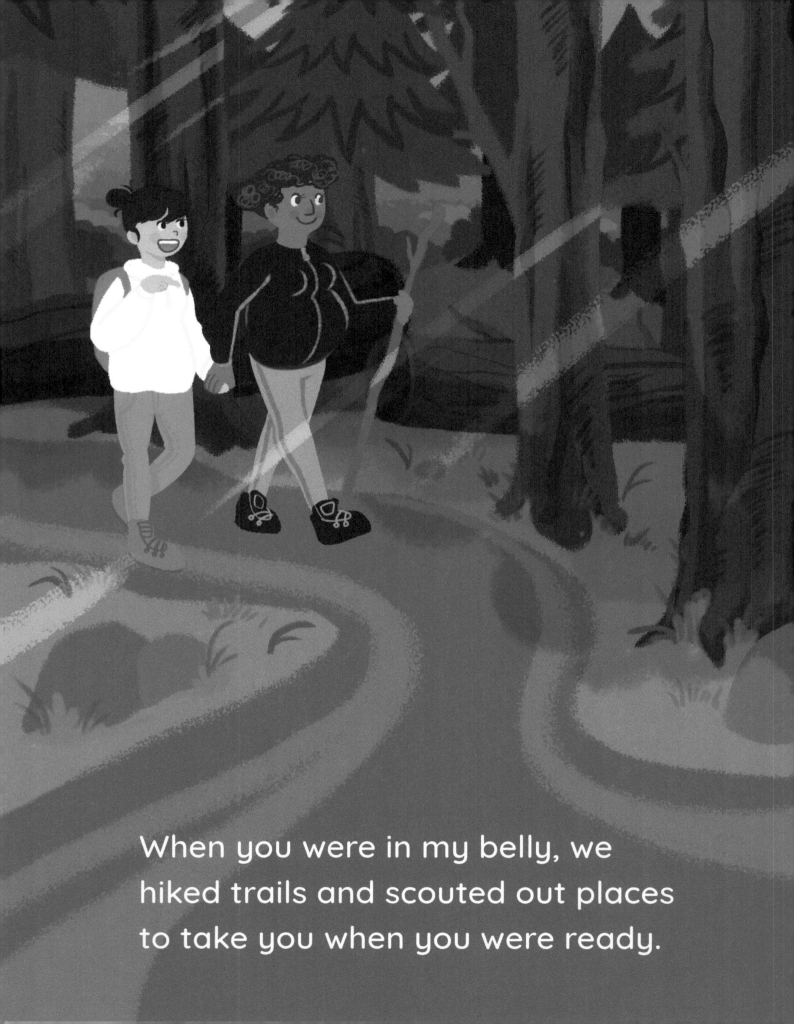

When you were in my belly, we hiked trails and scouted out places to take you when you were ready.

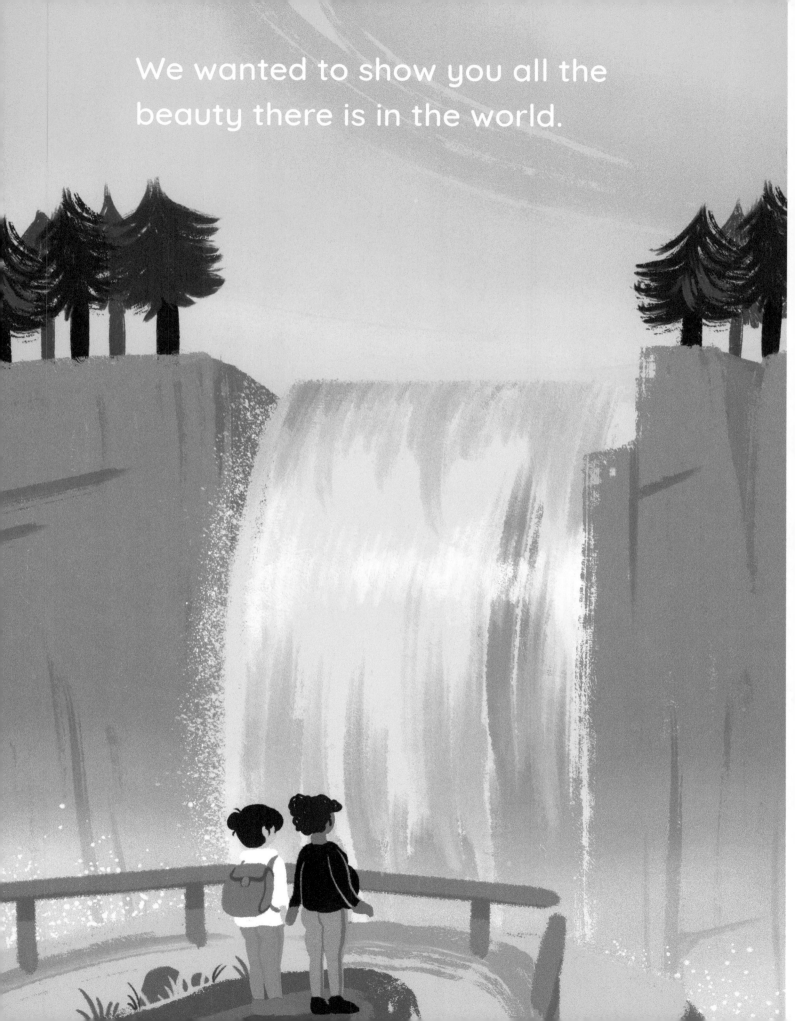

We wanted to show you all the beauty there is in the world.

When you were in my belly, we imagined a world where you would be safe, happy, and healthy.

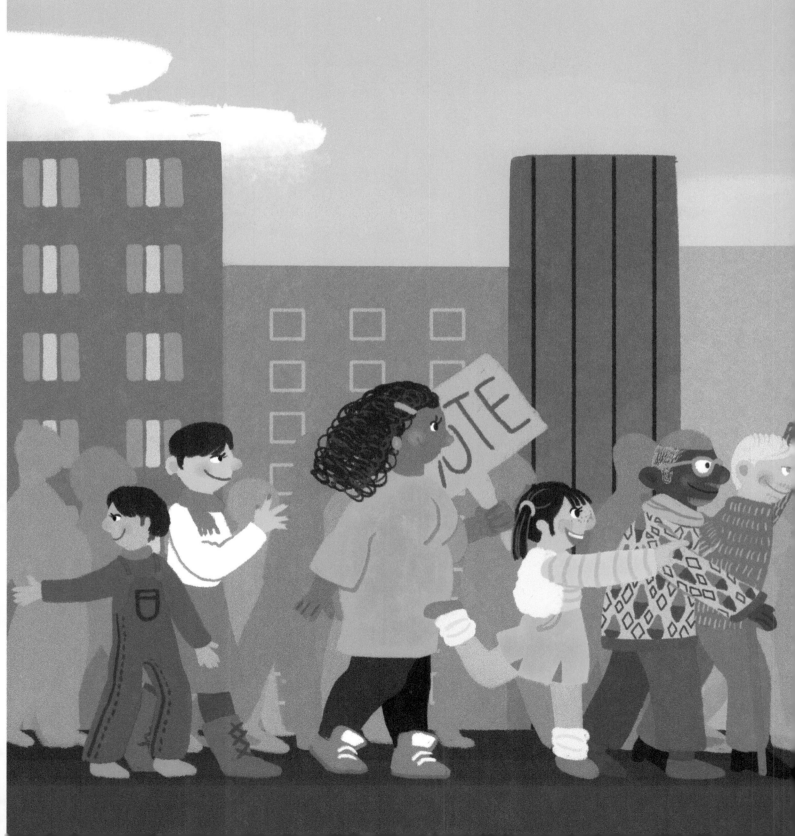

We marched for a better future for you.

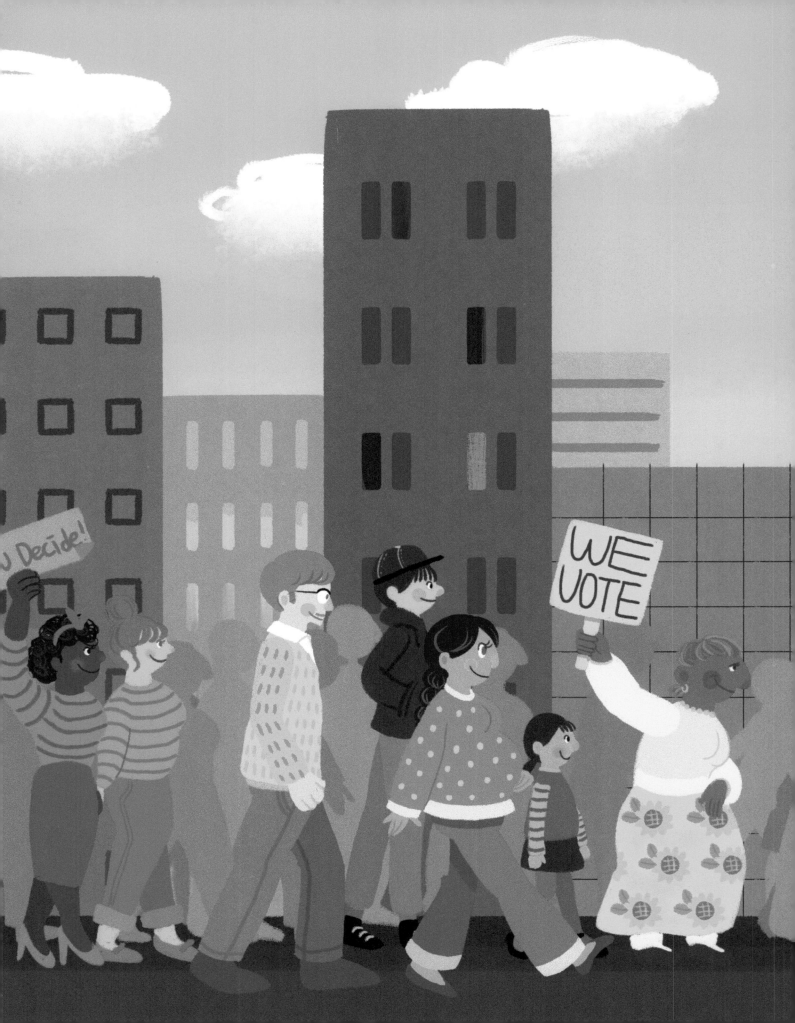

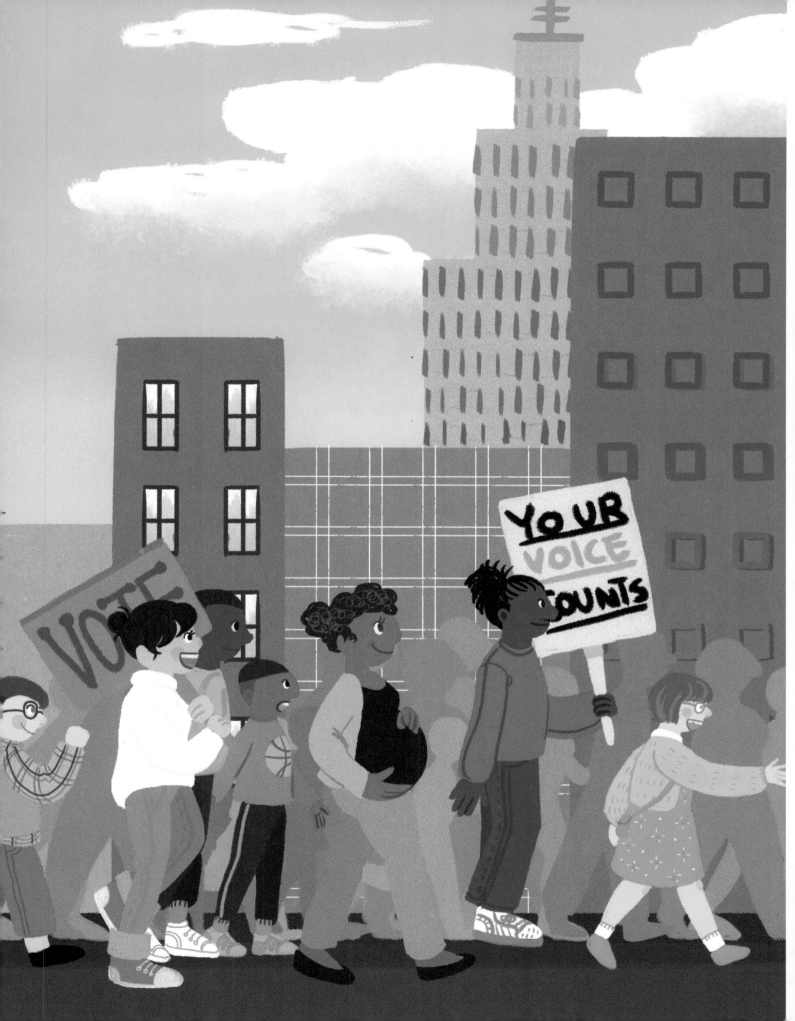

When you were in my belly,
we fell asleep with you
wrapped in our arms.

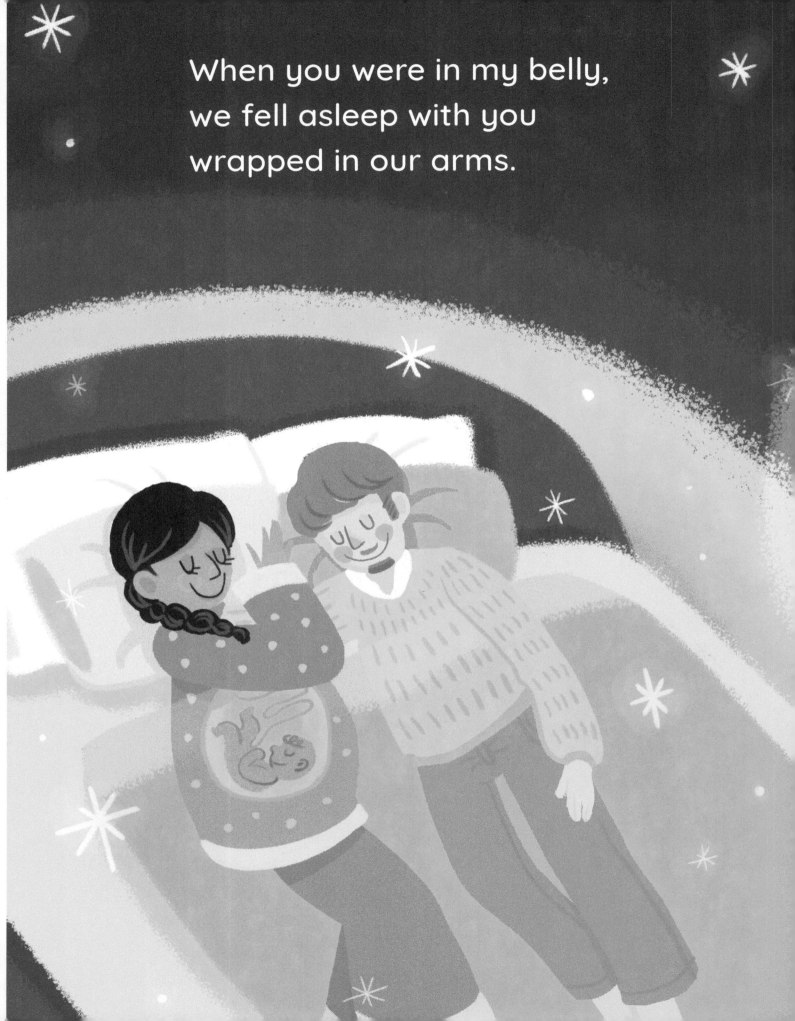

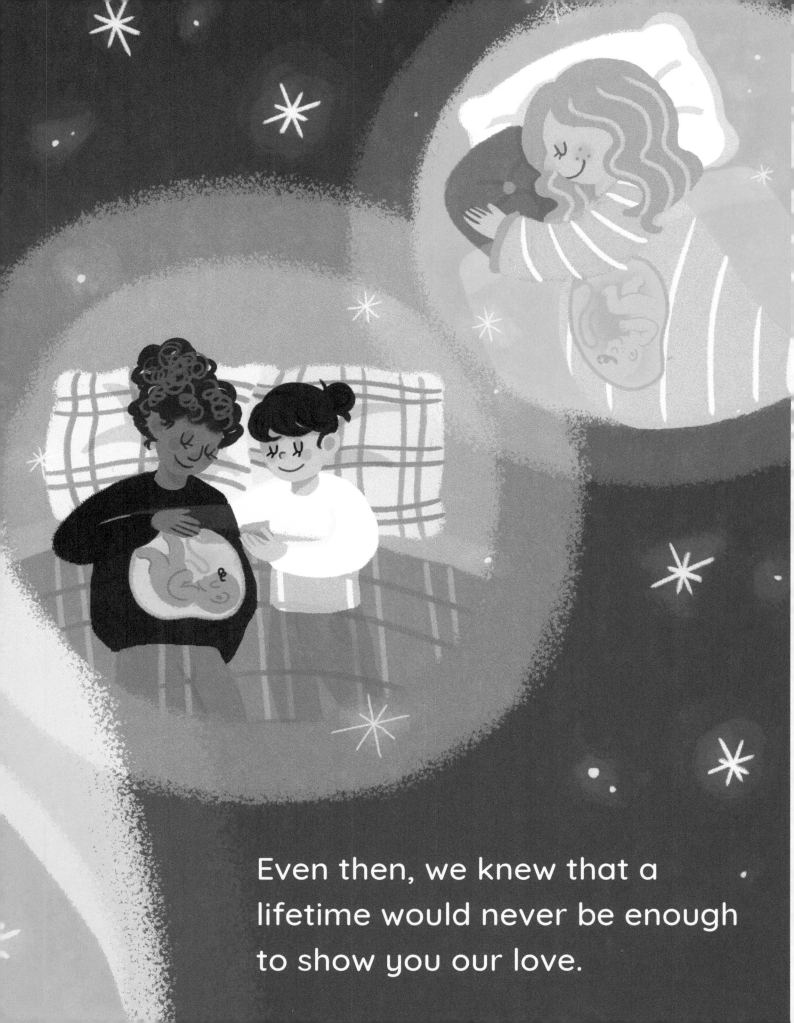

Even then, we knew that a lifetime would never be enough to show you our love.

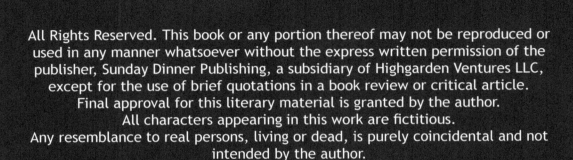

All Rights Reserved. This book or any portion thereof may not be reproduced or used in any manner whatsoever without the express written permission of the publisher, Sunday Dinner Publishing, a subsidiary of Highgarden Ventures LLC, except for the use of brief quotations in a book review or critical article.
Final approval for this literary material is granted by the author.
All characters appearing in this work are fictitious.
Any resemblance to real persons, living or dead, is purely coincidental and not intended by the author.

Visit us online at: sundaydinnerpublishing.com

ISBN: 978-0-578-75183-2

Library of Congress Cataloging-in-Publication Data is available upon request.

©2020 Sunday Dinner Publishing, Inc. Sunday Dinner Publishing

Publishing Credits

Sunday Dinner Publishing, *Publisher*
Seth Rogers, *Editor in Chief*
Angela Johnson-Rogers, *Creative Director*
Kara Michelle Liu, *Editor*
Mark Y. Liu, *Associate Editor*
Kevin Pham *Graphic Designer*

Tell Your Story Here...

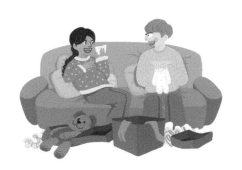

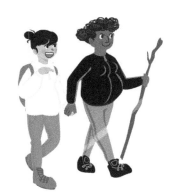

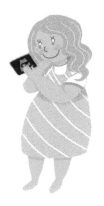

CPSIA information can be obtained
at www.ICGtesting.com
Printed in the USA
LVHW020605171220
674289LV00003B/49